Delayed But Not Denied:
The Journey of a Black Woman in Interpreting

By

Felicia P. Reed

Founder & Owner, Equivalent Communications

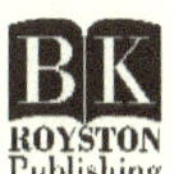

BK Royston Publishing
Jeffersonville, IN
www.bkroystonpublishing.com

Disclaimer: This is a work of nonfiction, while the stories and experiences shared are true to the best of the author's knowledge, some names and identifying details have been changed to protect privacy.

Cover design by Stitchwichs Custom Apparel & More

ISBN: 978-1-971868-19-6

Printed in the United States of America

Dedication

To my late father, Leo Reed, my hero, my guide, my anchor, and the foundation of the legacy I carry forward. Through your business Reeds Business Forms and Printing, you instilled in me the values of hard work, entrepreneurship, and integrity. I learned from you by absorbing your wisdom, work ethic, and love for building something meaningful. You paved the way for me, and I honor you by dedicating this work to your memory.

To Mrs. Donna Hawks, thank you for welcoming seven-year-old me into the world of American Sign Language and Deaf culture. You expanded my horizons, opened my eyes to a culture I had never known, and shared your knowledge with patience and grace. Thank you for welcoming that little girl into your home, your world, your culture, and for planting the seeds that have guided my lifelong journey."

Before the Journey

The First Book

Every journey has a beginning.

Before there was a career, before I was an interpreter, before I even understood the depth of what language could mean, there was a book. The very first book that introduced me to American Sign Language was *Learning American Sign Language* by Tom Humphries and Carol Padden. My mother kept it in our home, and one day she placed it in my hands. Holding that book felt like opening a door to a whole new world. At first, I didn't understand everything, but it sparked curiosity and excitement in me.

I didn't understand yet what this book was preparing me for. I only knew one thing; it was my mother who believed language matters. That belief quietly shaped the course of my life. Looking back now, I can see how the book revealed the beauty, depth, and expressiveness of ASL, and inspired me to keep learning, exploring, and growing in a language that connects so many lives.

So, from the bottom of my heart, Mama, I want to say THANK YOU! Thank you for your guidance, your discipline, and for giving me that sign language book at seven years old. Without it, I wouldn't have had the resource to study and grow in American Sign Language. You encouraged me to pursue my passions while ensuring I completed my homework and responsibilities first. Your wisdom, care, and structure gave me the foundation I needed to follow my dreams. I am forever grateful for your love and support.

This is my breakthrough book. It is a story of perseverance, faith, and the unexpected ways setbacks can become setups. It tells the truth about the journey, not just the destination, and it honors the process that unfolds when things do not happen on our timeline.

Within these pages, I share the resources, strategies, and lessons I discovered along the way, often in moments when I least expected them. I write honestly about the delays and disappointments, the season that felt stagnant, and the moments when I came close to quitting altogether. There were times when progress seemed invisible and the promise felt postponed, yet somehow those very delays became the training ground that strengthened me, clarified my purpose, and prepared me for what was next.

This book traces the years it took to get here, not as a list of milestones, but as a testimony of growth. Each season carried its own lesson, each setback revealed something necessary, and each disappointment required faith I did not always feel ready to have. Still, I kept going. Even when I doubted myself, even when the path felt unclear, I did not quit.

The tone of this book is encouraging, faith-centered, and deeply relatable. While I speak directly to interpreters and share experiences rooted in that world, this story is not limited to a single profession. It reaches anyone who has ever felt behind, overlooked, underestimated, or as though the promise was taking far too long to arrive. It is for those who have questioned their timing, their calling, and their worth while waiting.

This title carries God's timing written all over it. It is a reminder that delay does not mean denial and that what feels like a setback may actually be divine alignment at work. My hope is that as you turn these pages, you will see yourself reflected in the journey and be reminded that your process matters.

May you leave feeling inspired, encouraged, and uplifted, trusting that your breakthrough is unfolding exactly when it is meant to.

Table of Contents

Introduction

The Meaning of "Delayed but Not Denied"

I still remember the sting of those rejection letters. The bold black words, ***we regret to inform you,*** felt cold and final, as if they were quietly defining my worth. Each letter landed heavier than the last, especially as I watched others move forward while I seemed to remain in the same place. The messages felt robotic, impersonal, and dismissive, yet their impact was deeply personal.

Even in the face of repeated disappointment, I could not stop. I continued studying American Sign Language (ASL) relentlessly. I watched videos, practiced constantly, and immersed myself in the language whenever I could. At one point, I even taught an ASL class at a church in Nashville, Tennessee. That experience served as a reminder that this was not just an interest or a skill, but a purpose rooted deeply in who I was.

Life, however, had its own timing. After high school, I began college, believing I was moving forward, only for my path to shift in ways I had not planned. I became pregnant and married at the age of nineteen, and suddenly my journey looked very different from the one I had imagined. Still, even in those changes, God's hand never left me. I continued interpreting wherever I could, in schools, at work, and in everyday life. No matter where I went, my calling followed me. What I once saw as interruptions were actually confirmations that this purpose was woven into me, not dependent on a title, a position or a timeline.

These delays were not denials. Every challenge, every setback, and every pause was shaping me for what I was called to carry. Looking back now, it is clear that this journey was never about speed. It was about persistence, faith, and trusting that waiting does not mean failure.

This book is the story of that journey. It is the story of learning to believe that delayed does not mean denied.

Chapter 1

My Beginning: How I discovered American Sign Language (ASL)

I would come to realize that every setback, every delay, and every "no" was part of preparing me for the path I was meant to walk. It wasn't easy, and there were times I questioned whether I should keep going. But the language had already found me, the calling was already in me, and I couldn't ignore it. This is the story of how it all began. The first signs, the first lessons, and the journey that would shape everything that came after.

I was seven-years-old when my mother sent me next door to borrow sugar. In our house, it wasn't unusual to have peanut butter with no jelly, cereal with no milk, or one ingredient missing from whatever we were trying to make. Borrowing from a neighbor was normal.

What wasn't normal was what happened when I knocked on that door. I could see a woman inside, standing at the kitchen sink, washing something. I knocked once. She didn't answer. I knocked again. Still nothing. I remember thinking I know she can hear me knocking at her door. Finally, I rang the doorbell and that's when I noticed something strange. The light inside of her house flashed. A moment later, she came to open the door.

Standing in front of me was a woman with something bulky behind her ear, a cord running down to a black box clipped at her waist. Being seven-years-old, I did what seven-year-olds do best: I stared… and asked questions. A lot of them.

"What's that in your ear?"

"What's that box on your pants?"

"Why does your voice sound like that?"

She chuckled, kind and patient, and explained that she was Deaf. She told me that without her hearing aid, she couldn't hear anything. She also told me something that would quietly change the direction of my life forever. She said she communicated using a language. A language Deaf people use with their hands, to communicate, and it's called American Sign Language (ASL).

I was fascinated!

She explained that just like hearing people use their voices, Deaf people use their hands to communicate. It made perfect sense to me. When I ran back home, sugar still forgotten, I burst through the door and announced, "Mama! Our neighbor next door is deaf!"

My mother barely looked up. "Girl, I know that," she said. "Where is the sugar?"

I laughed, ran back and grabbed what I was sent for, then came back with a new request. "Mama, I want to learn ASL."

As it turned out, my mother already had a sign language book. At some point, she had taken a few classes herself. My parents made a deal with me: if I completed my homework every day, I could go next door to learn sign language. That was all I needed to hear. I didn't miss a single day. I studied the book at home and carried it back to Mrs. Donna's house, asking questions and practicing signs. She taught me patiently, answering every question I had. That was where it began. Curiosity turning into commitment, interest turning into love, and love turning into my passion.

When we eventually moved away when I was in middle school, life happened the way life does. I wasn't able to stay connected to Mrs. Donna like before, but the seed had already been planted. As I grew older, sign language kept finding me. At church, I joined the signing team and learned how to sign songs, such as *Jesus Loves the Little Children*, prayers such as *The Lord's Prayer,* and special programs under the direction of Sis. Tara. I learned that worship didn't have to be spoken to be felt. In high school, I attended a mainstream school with students of all abilities—Deaf students, blind students, and students using wheelchairs, all learning together. There were no separations or exclusions. It opened my eyes to a world bigger than my own.

I found myself watching the interpreters more than the teachers. I was captivated by how they took spoken words and transformed them into movement, meaning, and access. I wanted to understand and master that skill. I wanted to be part of that world.

Outside of school, I immersed myself even more. I attended Deaf events in Nashville, hosted by what was then known as The League for the Deaf and Hard of Hearing. However, the name has since been changed to Bridges for the Deaf and Hard of Hearing. The League for the Deaf and Hard of Hearing provided a safe space that felt welcoming, warm, and alive. I felt like I belonged. I then introduced and taught my family and friends sign language, signed with friends, and even interpreted informally when interpreters were late or didn't have a sub interpreter for my Deaf classmate. I didn't realize it then, but I was already walking in my calling and purpose.

At seven-years-old, I thought I was just borrowing sugar. I had no idea I was being introduced to the language that would shape my life.

Chapter 2

The Foundation Before the Calling

Before the word "interpreter" ever entered my vocabulary, my foundation had already been formed. It was rooted in faith, discipline, and purpose.

I was born and raised in church, and for me, faith was not an occasional practice or something reserved for Sundays. It was a way of life, present in every corner of our home and every moment of our family's routine. We attended services regularly at Greater Christ Temple Church (GCT), and we were there whenever the doors were open. Prayer was central to our household. We stood hand in hand in a circle, honoring God before leaving the house or beginning anything new. That consistent practice taught me order, patience, and reverence, principles that would sustain me through the seasons of waiting I would face later in life.

Entrepreneurship was another cornerstone of my upbringing. My father built his business, Reeds Business Forms and Printing, from the ground up, beginning in our basement on 600 Hamilton and later expanding to an office on Murfreesboro Road in Nashville, Tennessee. I watched him closely as he modeled professionalism. I watched how he dressed, how he communicated, how he treated people, and how he built lasting relationships. My siblings and I worked in the business from an early age, learning responsibility, consistency, and pride in our work. From him, I learned that excellence was intentional and that ownership required discipline.

Growing up in a two-parent household provided stability and clear expectations. Standards were established early, and values such as hard work, focus, and integrity were reinforced consistently by my father. Structure was never restrictive; it was grounding. It allowed me to develop discipline and resilience long before I encountered delays that would test both.

Nashville served as the backdrop for my early exposure to sign language and Deaf community spaces. I interpreted at church services, a community college, and in everyday interactions. Each of these spaces became a learning environment. I found myself drawn consistently to Deaf people, eager to observe, to engage, and to remain close to the language. I taught sign language informally when opportunities arose and made a point to stay present in every Deaf space I could access. I was hungry to learn, disciplined in my approach, and intentional about remaining close to the culture and the community.

At the time, I did not recognize these experiences as preparation. I only knew that I kept showing up. Only later did I realize that the patterns were already in place, that the foundation had been laid long before the calling became clear.

By the time I stepped fully into interpreting, I had already been prepared in ways I could not yet understand. Faith, discipline, purpose, and resilience had quietly shaped me, providing the grounding I would rely on for every challenge ahead. Stepping into this field as a Black woman would bring its own realities, layers of history, identity, and expectation that I had to navigate. The foundation had prepared me, but the journey ahead would test not only my talent but my resilience, my courage, and my belief in the value of my voice.

Chapter 3

Being A Black Woman in This Field

The patterns of my upbringing were already in place long before the calling became clear. At the time, I did not recognize those early experiences as preparation. I only knew that I kept showing up. It was only later that I understood resilience, faith, and excellence had already been woven into my character.

Stepping into the interpreting profession as a Black woman meant entering a space where very few people looked like me. I did not anticipate how deeply that reality would shape my journey. Being a Black woman in this field is not easy. From the very beginning, I learned that my presence alone invited assumptions about my intelligence, my skill, my professionalism, and my credibility.

I have been underestimated because of the color of my skin. I have been questioned because I looked young. I have been asked,

"Are you certified?" in ways that were not curious, but dismissive. I have been asked, "Can you really understand me?" as if my competence needed to be proven before I ever lifted my hands. I have even been told outright, "I don't want you to interpret for me because of the color of your skin." I never imagined I would hear words like that in a profession rooted in access, equity, and communication. But I did.

I was no stranger to being the minority. During my interpreter training program (ITP) in college, I was the only Black young woman in my cohort. I stood out whether I wanted to or not. One thing, however, remained consistent. I interpreted with excellence. Even without certification, I showed up as if I already had it. I prepared. I studied. I served. I took my role seriously because people's lives and educational access were never something I treated casually.

Still, it often felt as though I had to work ten times harder just to be seen as good enough, not only by members of the community, but at times by colleagues within my own profession.

One experience in particular nearly broke my confidence.

While working at a middle school back in 2010, I asked a colleague, a white woman, how she signed a particular concept. I expected collaboration. Instead, I was met with hostility. She said, "I'm not answering that for you. Didn't you just graduate recently? You should know how to sign that concept. You need to go back to college."

The truth was that we both held associate degrees. The only difference between us was that she was certified, and I was not. Her words cut deeply. They planted seeds of doubt I did not deserve to carry. Her name was Hannah, and in that moment I felt small. I felt unqualified. I thought, maybe I really do not belong here. Maybe I am not ready to be an interpreter after all.

What sustained me during that season was the presence of someone who chose to lift me up rather than tear me down. Her name was Mrs. Denice, a seasoned Black interpreter who became more than a colleague. She became another mother to me.

When I told her about my exchange with Hannah, she encouraged me. She mentored me. She prayed with me. She covered me. She helped me survive that school year. When I shared that I was considering going back to school to earn my bachelor's degree, she supported me fully. She told me about a University in Chattanooga, Tennessee, called Tennessee Temple University. The school is no longer in existence, but at the time it represented something powerful for me.

I was twenty-one years old when I packed up my life and moved to Chattanooga with my one-year-old son. That move was not just about education. It was about refusing to let someone else define my worth or my future. I remembered a professor once saying that in the coming years, interpreters would likely be required to hold a bachelor's degree. I decided to move forward rather than wait to be left behind.

There is a dangerous power in believing what others say about you when you are not rooted in who you are. If you are not grounded, someone else will gladly tell you who you are, and if you listen long enough, you may start to believe them. I learned that knowing who you are is not optional. It is essential.

Faith became my foundation. My identity in Christ became my anchor. Without it, I truly believe I would not be who I am today. No matter what I faced, I never stopped praying. I asked God daily to lead me and direct me.

Years later, life brought me face to face with the same colleague, Hannah. By then, I had experienced tremendous loss, including the death of my daughter, which required me to step away from work for a season. I was also going through a divorce. When our paths crossed again, I was interpreting at the very college where I had earned my associate degree.

She did not recognize me. I recognized her.

Still, I treated her professionally. I smiled. Gave her a tour of the campus. I showed her exceptional hospitality, as interpreters are called to do. I shared details about the student she would be covering in my absence. I explained classroom dynamics and expectations so she could provide excellence for the remainder of the semester.

Before leaving, I gently said, "Hannah, do you remember me?"

She said no.

I said, "Let me reintroduce myself. I'm Felicia. I'm the same interpreter you told back in 2010 that I wasn't good enough and needed to go back to college to learn ASL."

Her face went pale. The moment was quiet. Then she said, "Oh my gosh. Wow. How have you been? Do you think you can help me get on at this campus? I'm looking for work."

I smiled and replied, "If there are positions available, you'll need to go on the website and apply, just like I did."

That moment taught me a lesson I will never forget. Never underestimate people. Be mindful of how you treat others. Words spoken carelessly can echo for years.

I chose not to respond with bitterness, but I chose not to respond with bitterness, but I also chose not to forget the weight of what had been said to me. Integrity matters. Excellence matters. How we show up for others, especially when no one is watching, matters more than we often realize.

I remember calling my father and telling him what happened. I was upset. He said, "This is good." At the time, I did not understand. How could that be good? He said, "This is life. This is what makes you tough. Not everyone will treat you with kindness. However, you stay calm and you must remember to treat people the way you want to be treated no matter what. Keep going." I did not understand his words then, but I understand them now.

Confidence was not something I was born with. It was built over time. It was formed through preparation, consistency, and faithfulness when no one was applauding. It was shaped by staying connected to people who poured into me when I wanted to quit. People like Mrs. Denice. Mrs. Tena. Mrs. Donna. My parents. My brothers and sister. My entire family. And other people who prayed for me when my strength ran thin.

Discipline meant showing up fully even when I felt questioned, overlooked, or dismissed. It meant doing the work when I was unsure of the outcome. I learned to let my actions speak when my presence was challenged and to trust that faithfulness in small things would eventually lead to something greater.

Even when the destination was unclear, I kept showing up. I kept learning. I kept going. I learned that delay did not mean denial. But persistence does not mean the road was easy. It does not mean I avoided failure, loss, or moments where I questioned everything I thought I knew about myself.

What came next would take me places preparation alone could not. It would require more than knowledge, more than skill. It would demand obedience, surrender, and a kind of faith that survives when everything familiar is stripped away.

And that is where the real breaking began.

Chapter 4

Tests, Attempts, Failures, and Emotional Breakdowns

In June of 2018, I took a leap of faith with nothing but obedience and desperation holding hands.

I had lost almost everything. I was living with my mother at this time and my son and I were unstable. All I owned was a bed, a dresser, my 2007 Jeep, two hundred dollars, and a faith that refused to die even when it had every reason to. A friend from college connected me to his sister, Teresa, who opened her home to me and my son. That grace kept us afloat. Still, I made the painful decision to send my son back to Chattanooga to stay with his aunt while I tried to get on my feet. It was one of the hardest choices I've ever made.

Charlotte, North Carolina was unfamiliar territory. I had never visited or lived there before. As I drove from Nashville to Charlotte, mile after mile, I kept praying that

God would stretch that $200 and somehow, He did. I started at a truck company, working the window, handing slips of paper to drivers. I hated the job, but it paid $13.50 an hour, and pride had no place in survival. I knew one thing for sure: I was not going back home.

Grinding wasn't new to me, but in this season, it intensified.

Within weeks, I moved from the truck company to working as a teacher assistant at an elementary school. Somewhere between clocking in and clocking out, I was still dreaming, still believing, and trying to figure out how interpreting would fit into this new life I was building.

By July 24, 2018, I had the keys to a one-bedroom apartment in Fort Mill, South Carolina. It was small, but it was ours. For the first time in a long time, my son and I had stability.

A few months later, while scrolling through social media, I came across a post for a video relay company that was hiring interpreters. Video Relay Service (VRS) allows Deaf individuals to make phone calls through a sign language interpreter, using video technology. In a call center or a work from home setting, interpreters facilitate communication between Deaf and hearing callers in real time, relaying conversations back and forth, to ensure access and understanding. It was a critical service, and for me, it felt like a door opening.

I applied in November of 2018. By the end of that year, and into early January 2019, I began working as a Video Relay Interpreter (VRI). That opportunity marked a turning point. It was the first time my work aligned so closely with both my skill set and my calling, and everything began to shift.

I learned quickly that professional interpreting required licensure, discipline, and credentials. I did the work. I obtained my state provisional license. I accepted contracts. I worked at a VRS company. I kept saying yes to opportunities even when I felt underqualified, underprepared, or unsure. Eventually, I gave birth to my own business—Equivalent Communications—in February 2021. During the height of the COVID-19 pandemic, my business was nominated for Empowering the Carolinas. I received a $5,000 award, becoming the youngest recipient that year. I didn't win the grand prize, but I gained something just as valuable: confirmation that what I was building mattered.

And yet, behind the scenes, another story was unfolding.

I began taking certification exams. I studied. I prayed. I failed. I tried again. Some exams required more than one attempt, and others tested my endurance in ways I was not prepared for. Each failure cut deeper than the last, not because I lacked skill, but because I kept questioning whether this path was truly meant for me.

There were nights I cried until my chest hurt. Moments when I questioned whether this path was ever meant for me. Times when my own son became my encourager, reminding me of who I was when I had forgotten. I attended workshops, trainings, and seminars relentlessly. And eventually, I realized the noise was drowning me. I had to get quiet. I stopped chasing every resource and mentor and began studying alone. Just me and God. In silence. With discipline. With surrender.

Yet still, the failures came.

What no one tells you is that repeated failures can distort your identity if you're not careful. I lost myself for a while. I got distracted. I doubted. I broke down. And then, at my lowest, I stopped fighting and surrendered. I trusted that God had not brought me this far to abandon me now. I trusted that delay did not mean denial, even when my emotions told a different story.

The strangest part of it all was this: I kept showing up as if I was already certified. I served with excellence. I honored the work.

I stayed faithful to the call, even when the credentials lagged behind the calling.

By July 2025, it marked seven years since my son and I arrived in the Carolinas with nothing but faith, hope, belief, and trust. In Scripture, seven represents completion. I don’t believe that is coincidence. I believe seasons close when they have finished teaching us what we need to learn.

I believe seasons close when they have finished teaching us what we need to learn.

Chapter 5

Survival Seasons and Silent Persistence

By the time 2019 arrived, I was still finding my footing. I was raising my son in unfamiliar territory, building a career in interpreting, and trying to establish stability with limited resources and even less certainty. Like many women in survival mode, I made decisions rooted more in necessity than alignment. I believed that structure and partnership would help me manage the weight I was carrying, and for a season, I convinced myself that it was and that it was enough.

What I didn't understand at the time was that survival has a way of disguising itself as wisdom. I wasn't choosing from wholeness, but I was choosing from exhaustion. I entered a relationship that eventually led to marriage fairly quickly. I believed it would provide security and support during a fragile chapter of my life. While it served a purpose for a time, it became clear that it was not a sustainable fit. It wasn't about fault or failure. It was about misalignment. I was not the wife I needed to be and the life I was trying to build required more than I was capable of giving in that space.

By August 2023, I made the difficult decision to begin again. This time with intentionality, creating a home for myself and my son. What followed was not immediate peace, but a long season of emotional noise. Between 2023 and early 2025, I found myself scattered. I joined spaces, searching for belonging, connected with people who were not aligned with my healing, and overshared pieces of myself that should have been protected. I was trying to be everything at once: a mother, an entrepreneur, an interpreter, a woman of faith, and simply a human being who was tired of *surviving.*

From the outside, I appeared productive. I was still working. Still interpreting. Still attending workshops and trainings. Still studying. Still taking exams. Still saying yes to opportunities while feeling underqualified and overwhelmed. But internally, I was fragmented. I was healing and hurting at the same time. I was functioning, but I was not grounded.

There were moments during this season when I questioned everything. My calling. My identity. My resilience. I wondered where I belonged, who my people were, and whether the sacrifices were worth the cost. I tried different churches. Different communities. Different versions of myself. I said yes to rooms that drained me because I didn't yet trust my discernment enough to say no.

What no one prepares you for is how easy it is to lose yourself quietly. There is no dramatic collapse, just subtle erosion. Repeated disappointments, unmet expectations, and delayed dreams can chip away at your confidence if you're not careful. I was still showing up, but parts of me were unraveling.

And yet, through all of it, I did not stop pursuing interpreting.

Even when my focus wavered. Even when my heart was heavy. Even when I questioned whether I had the strength to keep going. I continued to take exams. I continued to train. I continued to invest in my growth. There were days I studied while emotionally exhausted. Nights I cried until my chest hurt, only to wake up and try again. Failure came more than once, but so did perseverance.

I almost quit during this season. Not loudly. Quietly. Slowly. In the way people do when they are tired of hoping. But something in me refused to let go completely.

That shift came when I was introduced to Improving Rural Interpreter Skills Training (IRIS) by way of University of Northern Colorado. For the first time in a long while, I felt like I belonged. I found myself in a space that didn't require performance or explanation. I was surrounded by interpreters who understood the weight of the work, the discipline it demanded, and the resilience it required. Through IRIS, I didn't just grow professionally, but I found my people.

What emerged from that experience was my KISS-TEA cohort family. We trained together. We struggled together. We celebrated small wins and survived setbacks side by side. Over the last two years, we have carried one another through moments when quitting felt easier than continuing. Their presence in my life was not accidental. It arrived exactly when I needed it the most.

What I learned about success is that it requires endurance. It is about continuing to show up when life is loud, confusing, and unresolved. I was distracted. I was hurting. I was searching. But I did not quit.

What I didn't know then was that God was preparing me for a season of redirection. One that would require silence, isolation, and clarity. A season where I would have to step away from noise in order to finally hear His voice.

That season would come next.

Chapter 6

When God Speaks: You Must Obey

After seasons of noise, distraction, and survival, God began to speak to me in a different way. It was quiet, firm, and without negotiation. This was not a season of explaining myself. It was a season of movement. God made it clear: be still, be silent, and obey.

One of the first acts of obedience was reclaiming my name. I returned to my maiden name, not just legally, but symbolically. It was an act of restoration of identity, of clarity, of grounding myself back into who I was before survival forced me to become someone else. Along with that came practical boundaries. I changed my phone number and became intentional about who had access to me. Not everyone needed my number. Not everyone deserved proximity.

I was learning, for the first time, how to protect my peace.

As a single mother again, I understood that guarding my home was no longer optional. My peace mattered. My son's peace mattered. I had to learn that access is a privilege, not a right. I began to understand life through circles—an inner circle, a middle circle, and an outer circle, and to place people where they belonged. These were tools I had not been given growing up. I learned them in real time, through prayer, discernment, and painful trial and error.

During this season, God instructed me not to announce my moves. In the past, I had shared too soon, testimonies still in process, instructions not yet fulfilled. This time, God said plainly: *move quietly.* There would be no explaining, no defending, no seeking validation. Obedience did not require an audience.

God planted me at Elevation Church in North Carolina, under the leadership of Pastor Steven Furtick. This was not about popularity or performance; it was about alignment. I was fed spiritually in ways I had not experienced before. Around the same time, I joined a divorce and separation support group which was something I had never done. I had always leaned on people who were not assigned to carry me, then felt disappointed when they could not show up the way I needed. This season taught me the difference between support and substitution.

God was rearranging everything.

As the IRIS program came to a close, I made one of the hardest but most necessary decisions of this chapter: I cut off relationships that were no longer aligned with my values, my morals, or the woman I was becoming. Some of these connections were familiar. Some were comfortable. But comfort without alignment is costly. Obedience required separation.

This was not easy. My son witnessed these changes. He watched me shed layers, routines, and relationships. In many ways, it felt like transformation happening in real time. It was slow, uncomfortable, and necessary. There were nights when I questioned myself again. *Did I make the right choice? Should I move somewhere else? Did I mishear God?*

But instead of moving me geographically, God redirected me inward, back to Him, and back to myself.

In this season, I learned a truth that reshaped everything: everything I needed was already within me, because God was my source. I no longer needed to pull from people what only God could supply. I realized how often I had looked outward for confirmation, reassurance, and security, when God had already provided it.

This was my seventh year.

When I first arrived in North Carolina, it was just my son and me. And now, after everything, it was just my son and me again. But this time, I was different. I could not afford to repeat old mistakes. I was older. Wiser. More discerning. My son was older, too, and I could see the fruit of obedience reflected in his growth.

My mornings changed. I stopped reaching for my phone first. I stopped checking emails, messages, or notifications before grounding myself. Instead, I reached for water, for stillness, for prayer. I got on my knees and asked God for wisdom, knowledge, and understanding. I learned to seek first the Kingdom of God and His righteousness, trusting that everything else would follow.

I could no longer live half in and half out. Lukewarm faith was no longer an option. This season required a decision to move forward without constantly looking back.

On July 11, 2025, in obedience rather than confidence, I made the decision to move forward again. I registered to take the National Interpreter Certification (NIC) exam for the third time, and the Educational Interpreter Performance Assessment for the second time in April of 2025. There were no guarantees, only faith. But this time, the decision was not rooted in desperation. It was rooted in clarity.

God was speaking.

I was listening.

And for the first time in a long time, I was moving in the same direction as my purpose.

Chapter 7

"Everything is Good. Everything is Fine."

I was at work, logged into my Video Relay Service shift. I was doing what I had done countless times before—interpreting calls, moving between silence and sound, waiting on hold. In the middle of an ordinary workday, an extraordinary email came through. It was from CASLI. The subject line alone stopped me.

CASLI: Performance Exam: NIC Exam Results

"Hello Felicia Reed,
CONGRATULATIONS! We are pleased to inform you that you have PASSED the Performance Exam for the National Interpreter Certification (NIC)!"

On December 1, 2025, I learned that I had officially passed the NIC Performance Exam. After years of preparation, setbacks, and repeated attempts, I was now a NATIONALLY CERTIFIED

INTERPRETER. A BLACK NATIONALLY CERTIFIED INTERPRETER AT THAT!

Seven years.

Three attempts.

Countless prayers.

Earlier that year, in April, I had taken the Educational Interpreter Performance Assessment for the second time. When the results came back in October 2025, I learned I had PASSED with a score above what was required. I needed a 3.5. I earned a 4.0+. This higher score assessment ensured I could continue serving Deaf and hard-of-hearing students in K-12 educational settings with excellence and credibility.

Acceptance after acceptance.

Confirmation after confirmation.

And then, just days later, on December 5, 2025, my son, Devan, received his second college acceptance letter!

Congratulations had become the theme of the season.

Congratulations – You Passed.

Congratulations – You're Certified.

Congratulations – Your Son IS Accepted.

Everything I had been working toward in silence was now being spoken aloud.

I called my dad.

I told him I passed. I then passed the phone to Devan so he could share his good news with his PawPaw.

My father cried.

That moment etched into my heart forever. My DAD. My coach, my encourager, my steady voice broke down in tears on the phone. He had watched this journey from the beginning. He had prayed with me. He had corrected me. He had reminded me who I was when I had forgotten.

My family celebrated. My community celebrated. My Tennessee people celebrated and those who had been rooting for me long before my credentials existed, before titles were attached to my name, and before the world could measure what God had already placed inside of me. They knew what this meant. National Certification wasn't just a professional milestone. It represented expanded access, increased opportunity, and long-term stability.

But more than that, it represented obedience rewarded.

My dad always told me, *"Whatever you do, stay humble. As quickly as the Lord gives you, He can take it away just as quickly.*" When I made mistakes, I called my dad. When I doubted myself, I called my dad. When I cried, my dad reminded me to lift my head up and keep going.

"If it were easy," he'd say, "everybody would be doing it." Those words carried me.

Then on Wednesday, December 10th, at 7:24p.m., my phone rang. It was my stepmother, Linda. My father had passed away.

Grief does not ask permission. It does not wait for joy to settle. It arrives abruptly, interrupting celebration with silence. My dad, my best friend, my motivator, and my anchor was gone. My father lived for seventy years. God allowed him to stay long enough to hear the words that mattered most: *"Daddy, I did it. I passed."*

As I reflect on the seven years since my son and I arrived in North Carolina with nothing but faith, $200, and a 2007 Jeep Cherokee, I see God's hand everywhere. Seven years. Three NIC attempts. Two EIPA attempts. Seven years of becoming.

My dad left me a legacy. Not just his business, Reeds Business Forms and Printing, but his wisdom, his scripture. His faith. He taught me to let go of the past, to stay focused, to keep moving forward even when my heart felt heavy. And now, when I look back over the journey, I can say with confidence, just as he always did:

Everything is good.

Everything is fine.

God allowed my father to see his baby girl, his "Granny", as he called me, make it. God allowed him to hear that I became a Nationally Certified Black Interpreter, equipped and authorized to continue serving Deaf adults and Deaf students with excellence.

I already knew what God had placed inside of me long before any exam confirmed it. But certification matters in the world we live in. It opens doors. It validates skill. And when preparation meets opportunity, it makes the journey sweeter.

This chapter is not just about credentials.

It is about legacy fulfilled.

It is about God's timing being perfect.

It is about finishing a race my father cheered me through.

And as I step into the next season, feeling grateful, grieving, and grounded, I carried his words with me:

Hold your head up high.

Keep going.

And always remember, Granny, that "Everything is good. Everything is Fine."

Chapter 8

New Confidence. New Clarity. A New Season.

December 2025 had already taken so much from me. I had celebrated. I had grieved. I had buried my father. And then, on Christmas Eve, it demanded something else from me.

I was leaving work, planning to stop at Honey Baked Ham to pick up dinner for the holiday, when my 2007 Jeep, faithful through over 338,000 miles, made a final decision for me. That car had carried me through survival seasons, through moves, through exhaustion and hope. It said, *no more.*

For a moment, the weight of grief and responsibility settled over me. I wondered, Lord, how am I going to do this now? Two days later, the dealership confirmed what I already knew. The Jeep was beyond repair. It was too old, it had too many miles, and it was not wise to fix it.

I thought about my son, soon leaving for college. I thought about the responsibilities ahead of me. And then I remembered something my father always said: *Everything is good. Everything is fine.*

On Saturday, December 27, 2025, I went back to the dealership. I took an Uber, but I was clear. I could not leave without a vehicle. I did not need luxury. I did not need excess. I needed reliability, safety, something that could carry me and my son through the next seasons. That was when God showed me again that provision does not always look the way we imagine, but it always arrives right on time.

I drove off in a 2025 white Nissan Altima. Reliable. Practical. Steady. And then something stopped me in my tracks. As I explored the car's settings, I noticed an iPhone already connected to the system. The name on the screen was Leo. My father did not even own an iPhone. I sat in silence, not fearful, not emotional in the way I might have expected, but assured, calm, covered, and seen. I refused to delete it.

I named my car Angel. She is white, dependable, carrying us safely, just like an angel. Whether anyone else understands it or not, I know in that moment God and my father reminded me. You are not alone. You never have been.

This season of my life feels different. I feel confident, not loud, not performative, but settled confidence. I know my vehicle will get me to where I need to go. I know I can show up to my interpreting assignments safely. I know I am no longer scrambling.

At the same time, I began clearing spaces. Garbage bags full of old things, clothes, papers, items, left my home, and in the same rhythm, they left my spirit. I shed a version of myself that no longer fit. And then LaShawnda entered my life.

LaShawnda is my yoga instructor and she became so much more than that. She taught me how to grow from the inside out. She taught me to breathe through tension, not shallow, but deep, intentional breaths that met the body exactly where it was. She taught me how to notice sensations I had been ignoring, the cold against my skin, the heaviness in my jaw, the tightness in my chest, and to simply hold and release them.

Through her guidance, I realized that stillness is not weakness. Reflection is not failure. To simply be is not laziness. It is preparation. It is a quiet power that comes before decisive action.

I realized something profound. I was no longer surviving. I was living. I was at my homeostasis.

God had put me back at the start line, but this time I was not the same woman who arrived seven years ago. I carried wisdom, discernment, boundaries, and lessons that I could not afford to ignore or repeat. I watched God remove people, strip distractions, and shed layers for me like a caterpillar becoming a butterfly. I trusted that what lay ahead was greater than anything I left behind.

I am grateful for forgiveness. I am grateful that God taught me how to forgive myself. I am grateful that I finally learned how to love myself the way He does. Everything I needed had already been inside me. LaShawnda helped me feel it. My yoga mat became a place of practice, a posture for life. Each exhale released grief. Each inhale welcomed clarity. Each session reminded me that God had me, I had me, and that was enough.

This chapter is not about the car. It is not about yoga sessions. It is about provision. It is about peace. It is about standing firm and realizing I made it through. I am steady now. For the first time ever, I am not rushing. I am not grasping. I am not proving anything.

My son witnessed the transformation. He saw me slow down. He saw me breathe. He saw me choose peace over panic, presence over performance. Without many words, he watched me become grounded, intentional, and secure in who I am. Children may not understand all the details of our journeys, but they feel the atmosphere. He felt the calm in our home, the safety of consistency, and the difference that presence and peace make.

I realized that my healing was not just for me. It shaped the environment around me. As I learned to sit with myself, to be still, and to trust God more deeply, I was also teaching my son what stability looks like. I was showing him strength that does not always need to be loud. Confidence that does not need to announce itself.

I was no longer surviving in front of him. I was living. I was steady. I was present. I was trusting. And this was the beginning of new season.

Chapter 9

Advice for American Sign Language Interpreters: Passing the Torch

This chapter is dedicated to those who are stepping into the field of American Sign Language interpreting, as well as those who have been called to mentor and guide the next generation. The journey of an interpreter is not just about mastering language, but it's about patience, perseverance, and serving others with integrity and compassion.

To anyone beginning this path, remember that your calling matters This work will challenge you, test your patience, and at times leave you feeling overlooked or underestimated. Stay the course. Every lesson, every setback, and every success is shaping you into the interpreter, the professional, and the person you are meant to become.

Learn from those who came before you, but also trust your own voice. Your experiences, your insights and your perspective are invaluable. Seek guidance when you need it, and remain teachable, but do not be afraid to step forward when the time comes. Growth requires both humility and courage.

For mentors, passing the torch means more than teaching vocabulary or technique. It is about modeling integrity, professionalism, and the faith and resilience that transform challenges into growth. Share your wisdom generously. Encourage your mentees. Create spaces where they can practice, stumble, learn, and rise without fear or judgement.

The beauty of this work is that it is not simply a career. It is a calling. You have the opportunity to touch lives, bridge worlds, and leave a legacy that extends far beyond the words you interpret. When you pass on your knowledge and encouragement, you clear the path for others just as someone once cleared the path for you.

Remember that your journey is bigger than yourself. Embrace your calling. Persevere with faith and pass on your knowledge and encouragement to those who follow. The legacy of an interpreter is not found only in skill, but in the lives you impact and in the torch that is faithfully passed to the next generation.

Final Chapter

A Promise Fulfilled

Looking back on this journey, I can now see how every setback, delay, and challenge was shaping me for what was to come. The tears, the doubts, and the long hours of studying and practice were all part of a greater plan. Nothing was wasted, and nothing happened too late.

Through every season, I learned that faith, persistence, and trust matter more than speed. Life may not unfold according to our timeline, but it always unfolds according to purpose. What once felt like delay was actually preparation. What once felt impossible became possible through obedience, perseverance, and the grace of God.

This book is my story, but it is also a reminder that your journey matters. Every lesson, every struggle, and every victory is shaping you into the person you are meant to become. If you are reading this, know that your path, however delayed or difficult, still holds purpose. Keep going. Keep trusting. Keep believing.

Your breakthrough is not only about achieving goals. It is about the growth that happens along the way, the resilience that is built, and the legacy you are creating. Every step you take and every challenge you overcome is part of a promise being fulfilled in your life.

As you close this book, I leave you with this truth that has carried me through every season. Delayed does not mean denied. Your journey unfolded exactly as it was meant to, shaping you, strengthening you, and preparing you for what is ahead. Trust the timing of your life and the purpose that is still waiting to be fulfilled.

Acknowledgements

To my brothers and sister, Leonard, Finesse, Kyle, and my twin brother Justin: I am deeply grateful for your love, support, and encouragement through every season of my life. You reminded me to keep going when I felt tired, to believe in myself when doubt tried to speak louder, and to silence the noise when the world became overwhelming. Your presence, your prayers, and your faith in me have been a steady source of strength, and I carry that with me always.

I want to especially acknowledge my Aunt Cora (Uncle Mason), Aunt Sandra, Aunt Sheron, along with my cousins George, Lauren, Courtney, and Charles. You have been an integral part of my foundation, showing up with unwavering support, wisdom, and love. I would not be where I am today without you.

A special thank you to my stepmother, Linda, for believing in me, investing in my growth, and consistently encouraging me along the way. Your thoughtful words, steady support, and timely reminders to keep going were meaningful nuggets that sustained me more than you know.

To my Kiss Tea family—Amy, Chelsea, Paula, Rochelle, Tammy, and Tina—your love and belief in me carried me through both challenges and celebrations. I am forever thankful for the community and encouragement you provided during pivotal moments in my journey.

To my yoga instructor, LaShawnda Lowe, thank you for teaching me how to ground, to breathe, grow, trust myself, and to simply be. You taught me the art of slowing down and embracing stillness in a world that constantly demands movement. During one of the heaviest seasons of my life, you became an emotional anchor for me. Through your guidance, you didn't just teach poses; you taught me how to breathe through discomfort, how to regulate my nervous system, and how to return to myself. The tools and practices you shared gave me real, tangible ways to calm my dysregulation and find balance again.

To Sis. Tara Jordan, thank you for allowing me to participate in the signing ministry (although technically we didn't have a name for it). You taught me how to sign The Lord's Prayer and songs like *Jesus Loves the Little Children*, moments that became foundational in my spiritual journey. I will always cherish the care and passion you shared each time you ministered. I noticed your body language, your facial expressions, and the love you expressed as you served, and I felt the depth of your devotion.

Being part of your ministry was more than learning signs. It was witnessing faith in action and experiencing God's love through your guidance. Thank you for giving me the opportunity to grow, to serve, and to share in such meaningful moments.

To First Lady Pamela Harris and the late Kena Coleman, thank you for welcoming me into the Anointed Hands Ministry. I am deeply grateful for the doors you opened and the space you created for my growth. Through interpreting, dancing, and serving in the ministry, I was able to learn, contribute, and grow in ways I will always cherish. Your guidance, support, and example paved the way for me to become the person I am today, and I am truly thankful for the opportunity to be a part of such a meaningful and transformative ministry.

To Mrs. Denice Simmons, from the very first day I met you, you exemplified what it means to be a true friend. When I was just finding my footing in the interpreting profession, it was you who coached me, disciplined me, and gave me at an early stage of my career. You stood up for me when it mattered most, and for that, I am forever grateful. From the bottom of my heart, thank you. I will never forget you.

To Mrs. Tena Spann, there are not enough words to describe the love and gratitude I have for you. You were not only my boss but a true friend, a guide, and a constant source of encouragement. You prayed for me and with me, covered me, cried with me, and even sat with me during the hardest moments of my life. You were there for me in ways that went far beyond work like looking after my son, supporting me through challenges, and always showing up when I needed you most.

Over the six or seven years I worked with you, you shaped and molded me, pushed me when I wanted to give up, and believed in me even when I didn't believe in myself. Your love, generosity, and unwavering support are a reflection of God's love in action. You exemplify it not just to me, but to everyone around you. I would not be who I am today without your guidance, your faith, and your example.

To Stitchwichs Custom Apparel & More, thank you for your loyalty, creativity, love, and unwavering support. Your belief in me, your friendship, and your commitment mean more to me than words can express. I am honored to work alongside you as my cover designer, and to witness the care, skill, and excellence you pour into your craft.

Everything you do reflects your heart and your love for what you create. You listen, you are attentive, and your creativity shines in every detail. I am deeply grateful not only for your incredible talent but also for the sweetness, generosity, and friendship you bring into my life.

I am deeply thankful to everyone who allowed me to use their homes, buildings, and churches as spaces to learn, teach, and practice ASL. Your generosity, trust, and openness provided me with safe and nurturing environments where I could grow my skills, explore my passion, and deepen my understanding. The lessons, experiences, and memories I gained in those spaces have helped shape my journey in ways I will never forget, and I will always carry that gratitude in my heart.

Sean and Teresa Stafford thank you both for believing in me when I was standing on faith alone. Sean, your encouragement and trust gave me the courage to take a leap I did not yet feel ready for. Teresa, your willingness to open your home to me and my son during one of the hardest seasons of my life provided more than shelter. You gave us stability, safety, and hope. Because of you, I was able to stand again. I will always be grateful to the Stafford siblings for the foundation you gave me.

To the Deaf Community, you have been the greatest teachers I could have ever been blessed with. You welcomed me with open arms, embraced me as if I already belonged, and shared with me your culture, your language, and your ways. You taught me the do's and don'ts, the consequences, and the importance of perseverance. You encouraged me, supported me, and cheered me on. You taught me about ethics, integrity, and what it means to serve with excellence.

Because of you, I strive to serve with excellence in every arena I step into. You stood by me through countless opportunities and through the times I stumbled and rose again. My becoming a nationally certified ASL interpreter is a milestone we achieved together. From the bottom of my heart, thank you for welcoming me into your world, for sharing your wisdom, and for allowing me to learn from you.

To my son, Devan, we made it! You have seen me sacrifice, cry, stumble, fall, and rise again. You have witnessed my journey to becoming a Nationally Certified ASL interpreter and an author. Thank you for your patience, support, encouragement, and for being such an incredible young man.

You are next in line as I pass this legacy to you. You are next in line as I pass this legacy to you. Everything I do, I have done for you, and I know you feel that in your heart. From the bottom of mine, thank you, son. I am honored and blessed to be your mom.

About the Author

Felicia Reed is a nationally certified American Sign Language Interpreter through the Registry of interpreters for the Deaf (RID) with over 15 years of experience across educational, religious, Video Relay Service (VRS), and community settings. She is committed to providing excellent interpreting and educational services, rooted in cultural competence, advocacy, and access.

She also holds a 4.0+ in the Educational Interpreting Performance Assessment (EIPA), administered through Boys Town National Research Hospital, demonstrating competence in educational interpreting settings. Her professional experience spans K-12, postsecondary and faith-based community environments. A native of Nashville, Tennessee, Felicia has been interpreting professionally since 2008.

Felicia's passion extends beyond interpretation; she is deeply committed to advocacy, access, and bridging communication gaps to ensure equity for all. This commitment led her to establish **Equivalent Communications** in 2021.

Felicia holds an associate degree in American Sign Language interpreting from Nashville State Community College, a bachelor's degree in management of human Relations from Trevecca Nazarene University, and a Master of Arts in Teaching Special Education from Liberty University.

To maintain excellence in her practice, Felicia regularly participates in workshops, trainings, and professional development opportunities, including completing the Improving Rural Interpreter Skills (IRIS) program.

www.ingramcontent.com/pod-product-compliance
Lightning Source LLC
LaVergne TN
LVHW050939080826
845145LV00004B/1329

* 9 7 8 1 9 7 1 8 6 8 1 9 6 *